CBD Root Guide

For PTSD, Cancer, Depression and More

By Chris Friesing

Introduction

Thank you for downloading this book, *"Cannabinoid Root Research: Benefits of Cannabinoid Roots"*.

Cannabis. Marijuana. So many other names but the reactions are the same- divided.

Some people treat marijuana as an evil weed to avoid. Some treat it as the cure they have been waiting for their whole life.

What about you?

What do you think of cannabis?

Is it a cure? Is it an herb that only seeks to destroy the mind?

This book will help you understand more about cannabis.

Here, you will learn what cannabis is. This is actually an ancient herb, used for treating numerous ailments.

Learn what makes this herb useful for treatments. Read this book to learn a whole lot more about cannabis.

Again, thank you and enjoy!

Table of Contents

Chapter 1

History Of Cannabis Use

Cannabis is an old herb, long been used for its medicinal properties. Several ancient societies have used this herb to heal or treat certain ailments. There are numerous mentions in the use of cannabis in ancient texts, which only proves that this herb does have therapeutic benefits.

Ancient China

The Ancient Chinese called this plant "Dàmá". The root word was "má", which meant "cannabis", "hemp" or "numbness". "Dàmá" also meant "big" or "great". In Taiwan, this plant was used for its fiber. The use of cannabis in these ancient societies started about 10,000 years ago.

Ancient Chinese texts described the plant, the parts, how to harvest, when to harvest, ho to prepare and how to use. The flowers are harvested after the pollen has been scattered. The texts recommend that the best time for harvest is on the 7th day of the 7th month. Seeds were gathered in the 9th month. Seeds that have fallen and covered with soil are no longer harvested. These will no longer be therapeutic and may likely be toxic, according to the Ancient Chinese texts.

According to ancient records, the first person to discover and use cannabis as an anesthetic was Hua Tuo. He was a surgeon c. 140-208. Hua Tuo turned the plant into powder form then mixed it with wine. This was given to the patient right before surgery. This is one explanation why the Chinese use the term "mázui" for "anesthesia". This word literally translates to "cannabis intoxication". These are just some evidences that as far back as 1st millennium BC, the Ancient Chinese already knew of cannabis' narcotic properties.

Furthermore, cannabis use was highlighted in the ancient medical texts called the pharmacopeia of the Tang. In these texts, the root of the cannabis plant was prescribed for blood clot removal. The juice extracted from the leaves was prescribed to combat tapeworm parasite infection.

Cannabis seeds were turned into powder then mixed with some rice wine. This form was mentioned in many other *materia medica* aside from pharmacopeia of the Tang. This form is recommended for numerous ailments, from hair loss to constipation.

The *Mingyi bielu* of the Ming Dynasty contained detailed instructions on how to harvest the heads of *Cannabis sativa*, which the Chinese called *mafen* or *mabo*.

A few ancient Chinese texts also had some reference to the flowers of the cannabis plant. Most of these texts agreed that the resinous flowering heads of the female cannabis plant were responsible for producing revelations and dreams. These texts also told of the effects of large intake of this plant part.

The *Shennong becaojing* is the most well-known ancient Chinese text with specific guidelines on using marijuana or cannabis for various treatments. These texts were written during the reign of Emperor Shen Nung.

The first record of cannabis root use for medicinal purposes was in the text *Shennong pên Ts'ao ching* (The Classic of Herbal Medicine). This was written around 2700 BCE, some believe to be around 2727 BC by the Chinese emperor Shen Nung. In this text, the root was prescribed as a remedy for pain. The powdered root was made into paste and used for fixing broken bones.

Traditional Chinese medicine listed cannabis as one of its 50 fundamental herbs. Every part of the plant was used for medicinal purposes. The flowers were recommended for treatment of 120 forms of diseases, including wound treatment and for menstrual disorders. The text is full of various recommendations.

Ancient Netherlands

Recent archeological findings found evidence that cannabis is also used as far back as 2459 to 2203 BCE, in northern Europe. A grave dated to be around the late Neolithic era was discovered in 2007. The grave had the remains of a peculiarly large amount of pollen. A five-year investigation found that the pollen were mostly cannabis. A small amount of meadowsweet was also mixed in. Meadowsweet has fever-reducing properties. Archeologists believe that this mixture was for fever and pain. The person in that ancient grave might have been very ill and cannabis was used as a painkiller.

Ancient Egypt

There were evidences that the Ancient Egyptians also used cannabis as part of their healing methods. In the Ebers Papyrus (dating back to 1550 BC), a prescription for medical marijuana was written. The cannabis was to be applied directly to control inflammation.

There were a few more Ancient Egyptian texts that mentioned cannabis. Examples were the Ramesseum III Papyrus (dating back to 1700 BC), Berlin Papyrus (dating back to 1300 BC) and Chester Beatty Medical Papyrus VI (dating back to 1300 BC).

Ancient India

Cannabis had a large part in Ancient India's medicinal and religious practices. Surviving texts mentioned about the psychoactive properties of cannabis. the Ancient doctors used these properties for healing. They used it for gastrointestinal disorders, pain, headaches, childbirth, and insomnia. It was also used for sunstroke, dysentery, to "freshen the mind", improve appetite, and clear phlegm.

Ancient Greece

Cannabis in Ancient Greece was used for both human and veterinary medicine. Sores and wounds on their horses were treated with cannabis. Dried leaves were used on humans to treat nosebleeds. The seeds were used in treating parasitic worms in the digestive system, such as tapeworms.

Pain and inflammation from ear obstruction were treated with wine or water infused with cannabis seeds.

Medieval Islamic world

Cannabis was used by Arabic physicians for various ailments. They used it as diuretic, antipyretic, analgesic, antiepileptic, antiemetic and anti-inflammatory. *Cannabis sativa* was used extensively in the medieval Islamic world for medications between the 8th and 18th centuries

Chapter 2

Types of Cannabis

There are two main strains of cannabis cultivated around the world: *Cannabis sativa* and *Cannabis indica*.

C. sativa

The sativa variety originally grew in areas near the equator. This is one of the oldest varieties cultivated for various reasons. This variety can be used for its seed oil and hemp fiber. People used *C. sativa* for food, for medicinal purposes, and even for recreation.

This strain primarily affects thoughts and feelings. The *C. sativa* strain stimulates feelings, making it a preferred strain for use during daytime.

Some of the known therapeutic effects of *C. sativa* use include:

- Stimulates or energizes

- Increases appetite

- Elevates mood

- Reduces depression

- Enhances creativity, focus, and overall well-being

- Relief from migraines, headaches, and nausea

C. sativa may cause some side effects, such as:

- Paranoia

- Anxiety

C. indica

The indica variety originally grew from areas in the northern latitudes. It is bushier and shorter than *C. sativa*.

This strain mainly affects the body. It has a tendency to produce feelings of sedation, making it a preferred strain for nighttime use.

Some of the known therapeutic effects of *C. indica* use include:

- Reduces stress

- Provides relaxation

- Reduces inflammation and pain from migraines and headaches

- Relaxes muscles

- Relieves spasms

- Helps improve sleeping patterns

- Stimulates appetite

- Reduces nausea

- Reduces anxiety

- Reduces seizure frequency (anti-convulsant)

- Reduces intra-ocular pressure

A few side effects have been noted with the use of this cannabis strain:

- Body malaise

- "Fuzzy" thinking

Cannabis ruderalis

This is a rare variety. The *C. ruderalis* is a variety native to Russia. The flowering period is earlier than the other two, more common cannabis varieties. This is also a stronger strain, able to withstand the harsher growing conditions.

Ruderalis is not popular choice. This strain contains low concentrations of THC compared to the other two strains.

With the recent findings on THC and CBD, ruderalis is now increasingly being grown because of its low THC content.

Hybrids

Aside from *C. sativa* and *C. indica*, there are hybrid strains. These are more commonly available than pure *C. indica* or *C. sativa*.

In these hybrids, one of the major cannabis strains is typically dominant. The characteristics of the dominant strain are usually the basis for determining the potential use of the hybrid.

For example, a hybrid characterized as a sativa-dominant cross may help in relaxing muscle spasms and increasing appetite.

Crosses or hybrids are effective as anti-nausea options and appetite stimulants.

All of these types have similar effects. These show potentials in reducing nausea and pain, improving muscle spasm, stimulating appetite, promoting better sleep, and so on. However, the degree of effects would vary among the strains because of the differences in the concentrations and ratios of the biologically active compounds. This is one reason some people find a particular strain more effective for a particular ailment than the others.

Chapter 3

Forms of Cannabis

Cannabis is not just about smoking rolled buds and leaves. It is now available in various forms. These forms, such as the oil, are better than the traditional smoking method. For instance, it is easier to control dosages with cannabis oil. Cannabis creams enable for more targeted treatment, limiting also the potential side effects or negative reactions.

Cannabis oil

This is also known as *cannaoil*. This is a cannabinoid-infused cooking oil. Several methods are used to create *cannaoil*. Cannabis and oil are mixed in a slow cooker, double boiler, frying pan, or pot. The mixture is heated gently over low temperature. The plant materials are strained out and the oil is now ready for use.

Cannabis oil has many uses. It can be a substitute to most oils in any recipe as long as cooking temperature does not exceed 280° F. This is the evaporating point of cannabis oil.

Examples of uses include candies, cookies, and cakes.

Tincture

This form is made by using ethanol alcohol for extracting the cannabinoids. Do not use rubbing alcohol. Choose pure grain alcohol or equivalent.

Tinctures are used in much smaller amounts than the other forms of cannabis. Use only in droplet amounts, administered directly into the mouth. Tinctures are easily and rapidly absorbed once it reaches the oral mucus membranes.

Spray

This is another method of using tinctures. The cannabinoids are still extracted from the glandular trichomes by mixing with ethanol alcohol. The product is applied under the tongue via a spray pump dispenser.

Cannabis liquor

Cannabinoids may be infused in liquor. Leaves and stems are the best used for making this form of cannabis. The plant parts are cooked into rum or brandy. A few drops of cannabis liquor may be added to beverages such as tea or coffee.

Cannabis topical

This form is applied directly onto the skin. The cannabinoids are mixed with a topical cream that easily penetrates the skin and the body tissues. Topical forms allow for direct treatment of affected areas.

This form is most preferred for conditions such as post herpes neuralgia, muscle or skin swelling, allergic skin reactions, inflammation (of skin and/or muscles), and muscle strain.

Pharmaceutical Cannabis or Cannabinoids

These forms have already been standardized in dose, formulation, and composition. Each spray or pill comes with exact and consistent amount of active compounds. These were developed following regulatory requirements. Pharmaceutical cannabinoids are prescribed by physicians.

These two are the available pharmaceutical cannabis:

- Dronabinol (Marinol®)

This is a prescribed capsule form of cannabinoids. Dronabinol is classified as a Schedule III drug.

This is typically used by patients after undergoing chemo therapy. Dronabinol is used for treating nausea and vomiting related to chemo sessions. This is also used in correcting weight loss and loss of appetite in patients with AIDS (acquired immunodeficiency syndrome).

Dronabinol contains a synthetic version of THC. This compound forms a suspension in sesame oil. This drug does not have any other cannabinoids such as CBD, only synthetic THC.

- Sotivex®

This is a prescription oromucosal spray. This is used for relief of symptoms of cancer and MS. It can help relieve neuropathic pain, overactive bladder, and spasticity, among others.

The active components of this pharmaceutical cannabinoid are extracted from two cannabis strains. The major active compounds are CBD and THC. These cannabinoids are mixed with ethanol to form a suspension. Each spray delivers a constant dose of 2.5 mg CBD and 2.7 mg THC.

Cannabis butter

Cannabis butter or *cannabutter* is cannabinoid-infused butter. Raw cannabis is heated with butter to extract the cannabinoids and mix it with the fat. Raw cannabis and butter mixture is heated at a low temperature in a pot, slow cooker, frying pan or double boiler. The plant material is removed.

This infused butter may be allowed to solidify and stored in the refrigerator for later use. Any recipe that calls for fats like butter and oil may use cannabis butter instead. Just check that the cooking temperature does not exceed 280° F.

Cannabis edibles

There's a growing movement in consuming cannabis through various dishes. Cannabis can be combined with various types of food such as cookies, cakes, and dressings. It may be added to different beverages such as herbal teas.

Heating the concentrates and extracts is recommended before taking cannabis. This helps in releasing and activating the cannabinoid tetrahydrocannabinolic acid into its active form THC.

When ingested, cannabis will be subjected to the digestive processes. This will alter cannabinoid metabolism, producing a different type of THC metabolite in the liver. This metabolite may or may not produce significantly different effects. This will depend on the individual, and the type, dose, and method of preparation.

The digestive process will delay the onset of effects but will typically last longer because the cannabinoids are absorbed more slowly.

When using cannabis through food, remember that the cannabinoids are hydrophobic, fat-soluble oils. These will dissolve more readily in oils, as well as fats, and butter. Cannabinoids are also more soluble in alcohol than in water.

Several converted forms of cannabis can be used in creating cannabis edibles. These forms can be made from the concentrates obtained from flowers and leaves. Example is hash.

Potency depends on the form of cannabis used and the amount added into the edible. Typically, using hash results in a more potent dish than one made with leaf trim.

Chapter 4

Understanding THC

Tetrahydrocannabinol or THC is the major bioactive chemical in cannabis that produces the psychological or psychoactive effects.

What is THC?

THC is the first cannabinoid to be identified in cannabis. This has also gone more extensive research compared to CBD.

This is a major constituent of extracts from cannabis plant. THC is found in highest concentrations in the resin from the trichomes. These trichomes are found in abundance in the buds and leaves. Stems also contain trichomes, but only in smaller amounts.

THC has strong psychoactive actions. It is also intoxicating, even when taken in small amounts. THC can alter behavior. It may even cause a person to lose control. These effects are what made marijuana a popular as a recreation drug.

Despite these effects, THC demonstrated a few desirable therapeutic benefits. It has been shown to be as effective in pain relief as moderate-strength analgesics. It can also be an effective alternative treatment of symptoms of some serious diseases such as AIDS. THC is more popular as a natural treatment for relief of symptoms associated with cancer chemotherapy.

The effects of THC have been tested in numerous research and case studies, and many anecdotal reports further prove its therapeutic potential. Hence, for decades, there has been a continuous movement towards the legalization of marijuana for medical purposes.

According to the NIDA (National Institute on Drug Abuse), THC acts similarly to the way the body's own cannabinoid substances act.

How THC Works in the Body

The brain has cannabinoid receptors concentrated in areas associated with pleasure, memory, thinking, time perception, and coordination. THC attaches to these receptors, thereby activating them. This activation causes changes in an individual's memory capability, movement, coordination, concentration, thinking, and pleasure perception. Time and sensory perceptions are also affected.

According to NIDA, THC has a stimulatory effect of the brain cells. It triggers the release of more dopamine, which is responsible for the euphoric feelings following THC intake.

The presence of THC in the brain also interferes with memory processing. It alters how the hippocampus processes information and memory formation.

Aside from these, THC can also cause hallucinations. It can change a person's thinking process. THC can even induce delusions.

The average duration of the effects of THC is two hours. The effects of THC are generally felt around 10 to 30 minutes after ingestion. These, however, vary depending on dose, history of marijuana use, condition of the user, and other factors. In some people, the psychomotor effects of THC persist even after the "high" has already waned.

Side Effects of THC

Some people experience side effects with use of THC. These include:

- Anxiety

- Elation

- Tachycardia (increased heart rate)

- Recall issues with short-term memories

- Relaxation

- Pain relief

- Sedation

Studies found that these side effects may be reduced or prevented when taking THC with other cannabinoid types. Examples are terpenes and CBD.

Risks

The effects such as pain relief make THC a very popular choice. However, THC use comes with a few risks.

Aside from a few negative side effects, there are concerns about the following conditions that may arise from THC use:

- May trigger relapse of schizophrenic symptoms

- Impaired motor skills

- Impaired coordination for certain activities such as driving, which may last for about 3 hours after taking THC

In fact, marijuana use is second to alcohol use in substance-use related road accidents, according to the National Highway Traffic Safety Administration.

In younger people, marijuana use is also placing them at risk for some problems. This includes a few long-term problems as well, such as:

- Decrease in IQ

- Decrease memory capabilities

- Decreased cognitive abilities

These long-term effects are still under more research to establish if THC does increase the incidence of these conditions.

Another potential risk in taking THC is impaired fertility in both men and women. This has yet to be established, pending additional research.

One study conducted in the University of Montreal found that early marijuana use can affect teens' development. This study was published in the *Development and Psychopathology* journal in 2016. This study found correlations in smoking, marijuana and school performance. Smokers who started at the age of 14 had lower scores on some cognitive tests compared to non-smokers. The study went further and followed almost 300 students. Those who smoked pot had higher rates of dropping out of school. Those who started at an older age, around 17 years old, did not have these same problems.

NIDA also studied the effects of THC exposure at very young ages. The study included THC exposure before birth (from mothers who smoked pot during pregnancy), soon after birth (babies from mothers who smoked while breastfeeding), or during adolescence. These children had difficulties in specific memory and learning tasks when they got older.

Overdose on THC

A small amount of THC can already produce intoxication and a few negative side effects. Hence, there is also the risk for overdosing on THC.

One of the growing concerns in the states with laws allowing marijuana use is overdosing on edibles.

People may have the tendency to eat more than the recommended small amount. For instance, one cookie made with marijuana may contain large amounts of THC. Eating one cookie may be enough to cause an overdose.

Edibles tend to have extremely high potency. When ingested, THC tends to last longer in the body. The effects may also last longer. This can turn into a serious problem.

The effects from inhaling THC typically last for about 45 minutes to around a few hours. For edibles, the effects can last for 6 to 8 hours. A single marijuana-laced cookie can quickly turn into a trip to the emergency department.

THC concentrations in cannabis

Another thing to consider about THC is air exposure. Exposure to air causes a chemical reaction that transforms THC into cannabinol. This is another cannabinoid that produces its own set of psychological effects.

Concentration of THC differs among the strains of cannabis. The lowest concentration is found in hemp. There is only about 0.5% THC in this strain. Hemp is more commonly cultivated for industrial and commercial use. It is not used for recreational purposes because of its lack of THC for psychoactive effects.

Chapter 5

Understanding CBD

A cannabinoid, CBD is a naturally occurring substance found in the cannabis plant. The roots contain the highest concentration of CBD compared to the rest of the plant.

Recently, this compound has been receiving much attention for numerous reasons.

CBD is one of the newer food supplements. It offers an impressive list of therapeutic benefits. Sounds like any other food supplement, right?

Knowing where CBD comes from makes this substance controversial.

CBD is extracted from cannabis or marijuana plant.

This is where the hot debates and widely differing opinions come in.

Therapeutic benefits of Cannabidiol

The list of benefits from CBD are mainly from reports of users. There have been several researches conducted to prove CBD benefits but have yet to yield conclusive evidences.

According to reports, CBD helps in relaxing both mind and body. It produces a calming effect that helps combat stress and anxiety. This compound is also a powerful antioxidant.

CBD is also effective in counteracting the effects of THC. Taking CBD can help address the "high" from THC. For example, a person experiences the "munchies" after taking too much THC. The increase in appetite may not be desirable for the person who took THC. To counter this effect, CBD is administered.

Source of CBD

As previously mentioned, CBD is one of the biologically active compounds in cannabis. It is one of the isolated and identified 85 different cannabinoids. This is the second largest substance in cannabis extracts, in terms of abundance. Cannabis extracts would typically contain up to 40% CBD.

The same extract would also typically contain THC, the psychoactive component of cannabis.

Unless, the source is the roots.

The buds and the leaves have high THC content, along with CBD. The stems also have a large concentration of these two. Only the roots have the highest CBND and almost negligible THC contents.

Effects of CBD

CBD does not produce the "high" or euphoric symptoms associated with marijuana use, even if taken in high concentrations. CBD products from the roots contain traces of THC, not enough to give the psychoactive effects. CBD-high hemp can be ingested or smoked in large amounts without experiencing "high". It is also almost impossible to get high with CBD oil and oil products that contain almost no THC. Nonetheless, CBD will still be able to produce the therapeutic effects such as pain relief and calming effects.

CBD is typically extracted as oil. It is diluted in hemp seed oil for easy dosing. CBD oil diluted in hemp seed oil is available in different concentrations.

Legality

With the growing research-based and anecdotal evidences, CBD is considered legal worldwide. Only Canada considers CBD as a controlled substance.

The hesitation about CBD is mainly from misunderstanding its chemical properties. It is also closely related to THC, which makes some people think these two substances are essentially the same. In fact, some people considered CBD as a precursor of THC. This caused some states to consider CBD as a controlled substance since THC is a strictly regulated substance.

Recent studies have given light on the CBD issue. Now, CBD is no longer considered a controlled substance in the same degree as THC. CBD is legal and can be safely consumed in any concentration or amount.

Chemical properties

CBD has partial resemblance to THC. However, the chemical chains of these two substances are completely different. THC and CBD are formed via different pathways.

How CBD works

CBD is different from most of the other cannabinoids, especially THC. CD does not seem to interact direct directly with the body's cannabinoid receptors. THC directly attaches to these receptors and produce the effects. CBD seems to behave differently.

CBD or cannabidiol has low binding potential with the body's CB1 and CB2 receptors. It works by acting as an antagonist to the agonists of these receptors.

Simply put, CBD enhances the work of these receptors. It keeps the receptors working at optimum levels. This means enhanced binding with other cannabinoids, producing greater levels of therapeutic effects.

To gain a better understanding, read the following simple definition of terms:

- Agonist: These are chemicals that bind or attach to a receptor. The binding activates the receptor. Once bound, a biological response is produced. This action is like putting a key into a lock and opening the door.

- Antagonist: These chemicals work opposite the agonists. When antagonists bind to receptors, the function is inhibited. It's like putting a key in a lock and locking the door.

- Inverse agonists: These are chemicals that bind to receptors as agonists but produce the opposite effect. It's like a key inserted into a lock and opening it but results in closing the door.

Functions of CBD

Scientists are impressed with what they observe of CBD. They believe that CD has more to offer. So far, scientists have found the following CBD function:

- Increase the density of CB1 receptors, allowing for more binding sites for other cannabinoids.

- Functions as agonist of 5-HT1a receptor. It binds to this receptor, producing soothing and calming effects like potent analgesics but causing no side effects.

- Functions as CB2 receptor inverse agonist. This acts against cannabinoids that reduce CB2 responsiveness. By acting as inverse agonist, "anti-CB2" cannabinoids won't be able to bind with CB2. This clears CB2, allowing for more CB2-related functions and effects.

- Functions as antagonist of GPR55 receptor. This is a newly discovered element of the body's endocannabinoid system. The function of the GPR55 receptor is still under research. CBD appears to act as an antagonist to this receptor.

CBD vs THC

Both of these compounds interact with the cannabinoid receptors in the body. This ability allows them produce some effects that can be therapeutic.

The scientific community generally accepts CBD as safer than THC. A significant number of studies found a correlation between the long-term THC use and the development of psychiatric disorders such as psychosis, depression and schizophrenia.

It is equally important to understand that a correlation is not causation. That is, people taking THC may develop these psychiatric disorders but THC is not the root cause of it. One way to see this is that smokers carry lighters but not everyone who carries lighters is a smoker. People taking THC may develop psychiatric disorders but THC is not the cause of it.

Available research results showed no negative effects from CBD, unlike in THC. This is primarily the reason for CBD's worldwide legality. A few case studies and some research also showed that CBD could provide some protective benefits against THC's negative side effects.

CBD is not yet fully researched, certainly not as extensive as THC in the last several decades. There yet remain more benefits to be discovered from CBD. So far, it is accepted that CBD is a safer bet in obtaining the therapeutic benefits of cannabis without suffering any negative psychoactive effects like in THC.

Chapter 6

Cannabis Root Topical

Cannabinoids applied topically have been found to have no psychoactive effects. Inhaling or eating the medicine has risk for experiencing some degree of psychoactive effect.

Using as a topical agent is one way to get the benefits of cannabis without experiencing the cerebral euphoria caused by other administration methods like inhalation.

With the growing interest in using cannabis as topical agent, new and longer lasting topical delivery systems are being developed. Examples are tingly lubricants and long-lasting patches.

How Topicals Work

Relief and other therapeutic benefits are achieved through the binding of cannabinoids to the CB2 network. CB2 is a network of receptors are scattered all over the body. CB2 is activated when the body's own endocannabinoids bind with it. Phytocannabinoids such as those from cannabis (e.g., CBD and THC) may also bind to these receptors, producing the therapeutic effects.

Topicals would only bind with the CB2 receptors. The cannabinoids won't be able to bind with other receptors. This is why topicals do not produce a "high" like other delivery systems. Even large doses with high concentrations of the psychoactive THC will not be able to produce the euphoric symptoms.

The cannabinoids from the topicals do not penetrate deep enough to reach the bloodstream. These only go deep enough to reach the CB2 receptors.

However, there are exceptions. Transdermal patches are designed to deliver medications and cannabis into the deeper layers of the skin structure. The medication can reach the bloodstream. If the cannabinoids on the transdermal patches contain THC, psychoactive effects may be experienced. The intensity of the psychoactive effects will depend on the concentration of the THC in the patches.

Therapeutic Benefits of Topicals

Poultice

The cannabis root poultice can be used for the following disorders:

- Cuts

- Dermatitis

- Burns

Balms, oils and salves

- Chronic larynx inflammation
- Migraines
- Headaches
- Tension pains
- Dysmenorrhea
- Acne
- Pimples
- Blisters
- Herpes
- Hemorrhoids
- Sore throat
- Asthma
- Colds
- Arthritis

Forms of Cannabis Topicals

Cannabis topicals come in various forms, such as:

- Salve

This is made by heating cannabinoids and coconut oil. The mixture is strained and mixed with beeswax. After the salve has cooled, it can be rubbed directly on the skin, over the affected area.

- Cream

The cannabinoid is combined with Shea butter then heated gently with a few other ingredients. The mixture is cooled before rubbing on the skin, directly over the problem area.

These topicals have analgesic and anti-inflammatory affects that relieve pain. However, recent research on the effectiveness of cannabis topicals is limited to post herpes and allergic skin reactions, as well as pain relief.

Other anecdotal reports on treatment potential of topical form include:

- Balm for lips, herpes, fever blisters

- Some types of dermatitis such as atopic dermatitis

- Psoriasis

- Superficial cuts, wounds, corns, furuncles, certain nail fungi infection, acne pimples

- Torticollis, muscular pains and cramps, back pains, sprains, and other contusions

- Rheumatism and arthritic pains (may help up to 2nd degree arthritis)

- Venous ulcerations, phlebitis

- Hemorrhoids

- Asthmatic problems with breathing

- Cold bronchitis, sore throat

- Chronic inflammation of larynx (application of cannabis through a Priessnitz compress)

- Migraine, tension headaches, head pains

- Menstruation pains

Chapter 7

Uses Of Cannabis Roots

The first record of root use was about 5,000 years ago, in ancient Chinese medical texts. According to these ancient literatures, cannabis root juice was used as a diuretic. This was also used in Ancient China on women to stop hemorrhage after giving birth. Other ancient Chinese literatures also documented the use of the plant as an ingredient in creating gunpowder.

In Ancient Rome, Pliny the Elder also made references about cannabis. This Roman Historian wrote in his *Naturalis Historia* about cannabis root boiled in water. This mixture was used as treatment for gout, joint stiffness, and related disorders. The raw hemp root was also applied on burns for soothing relief.

Manuscripts found in Azerbaijan dated from 9th to 18th century CE had references about cannabis roots. Decoctions were made and used for treating fevers and wounds. The locals in Azerbaijan used the cannabis root for abscesses, ulcers, and toothaches.

From this period onwards, very little literatures have any further mention of cannabis root. However, in recent years, there have been a resurgence in the interest and actual use of cannabis roots.

Contents of Cannabis Roots

The roots have little amounts of CBD and THC compared to the leaves and the flowers. However, the chemical analysis of the roots show that it contains bioactive compounds that produce some significant therapeutic effects. These compounds may provide the reason for the roots to be considered in the ancient times as an important herb for healing and for inflammatory relief.

Studies

The number of studies on cannabis as a whole is large but conclusive evidence is still lacking. Therapeutic claims are mostly based on anecdotal reports. The most commonly used plant parts are the flowers and the leaves. Not a lot of people know that the roots are therapeutic as well. Ancient texts do have references about health benefits of the root.

Available research results found that cannabis roots contain significant amounts of biologically active compounds known to have some positive effects on the body.

1. One study conducted in 1971 was able to find that cannabis root has several of the same terpenes found in the other plant parts. An astonishing finding is that some of the types of terpenes considered as minor in the rest of plant can be

found in abundance in the roots. An example is the compound friedelin. This compound has analgesic, antipyretic and anti-inflammatory properties.

2. Another research also found that there are significant amounts of alkaloids in the roots. This includes pyrrolidine and piperidine. These are valuable alkaloids in the pharmaceutical industries, being vital ingredients in many important drugs. The roots also contain choline and atropine.

3. Another study found that cannabis roots also contain spermidine. This can benefit those suffering from type 2 diabetes. This compound also showed some anti-aging properties that function at a cellular level.

4. A study conducted at Netherlands' Leiden University in 2008 found that the roots also contain glycoside. This is an organic molecule that can bind with toxins. This binding inactivates the toxins, which helps in cleansing the body.

Definition of Root Compounds

The roots are composed of sugars and lipids. Ethanol extracts of the cannabis root revealed that it also contains terpenes. Some of the important terpenes in the roots are:

- Friedelin

This acts as an antioxidant. It also exhibits protective effects on the liver.

- Pentacyclic triterpene ketone

This compound has been to effectively kill cancer cells. It may also decrease the severity of inflammation, combat bacterial infections, and promote diuresis.

- Epifriedelanol

This compound shows potentials in preventing tumor growth.

The roots also have a number of alkaloids, such as these:

- Piperidine

This is an alkaloid already used by the pharmaceutical industry in manufacturing drugs used in psychiatry.

- Pyrrolidine

This is another main ingredient used by pharmaceutical companies in manufacturing stimulant medications.

- Choline

In the body, choline acts as a vital nutrient in the maintenance of cell membranes. Choline deficiency in post-menopausal women may cause a few problems. Women may benefit from regular consumption of cannabis root tea to prevent this deficiency state.

- Atropine

It has a relaxing effect on the eye muscles. This may also help in increasing heart rates. Atropine also has bronchodilatory effects. It reduces the amount of bronchial secretions. It also relaxes the glands and the muscles controlled by the parasympathetic nervous system.

Chapter 8

Types Of Cannabinoids And Terpenes

Cannabinoids and terpenes are the active plant compounds in cannabis that bring the benefits and possible harmful side effects. Each variety of cannabis has different concentrations of these compounds.

THC is the first identified cannabinoid. This is also the most popular active compound. THC (delta-9-cannabinoid) has the most important psychoactive effect compared with other cannabinoids. THC ratio to other cannabinoid content varies among the different cannabis strains.

Other cannabinoids are non-psychoactive. The physiological effects of these cannabinoids have potential therapeutic uses. Examples of these non-psychoactive are:

- CBD (cannabidiol)

This cannabinoid has the same therapeutic qualities as THC without the psychoactive effects. CBD may be used to relieve inflammation, nausea convulsions and anxiety.

CBD is the main cannabinoid found in non-THC strains of cannabis. Modern cannabis breeders are developing strains that have higher CBD contents for use in medicine.

- CBN (cannabinol)

This compound has mild psychoactive effects. It may help decrease intraocular pressure and reduce seizure occurrence.

- CBC (cannabichromene)

This compound has analgesic effects similar to THC. This can be used for pain relief. CBC also has calming effects (sedative).

- CBG (cannabigerol)

This compound also has some sedative effects as well as antimicrobial properties. CBG may also help reduce intraocular pressure.

- THCV (tetrahydrocannabivarin)

This shows potential as a treatment option for type 2 diabetes and associated metabolic disorders.

There are other biologically active compounds aside from cannabinoids. Some of these compounds are terpenoids (or terpenes) and flavonoids. Terpenes are responsible for the smell, while the flavonoids give the flavor. These have a few therapeutic uses as well.

Cannabinoids, flavonoids and terpenes, along with other compounds are found in the hairy structures on the leaves, flowers and stems. These glandular trichomes (hair) secrete these active compounds. Trichomes are most dense on the flowers and the floral leaves of female cannabis plants.

Effects of Cannabis

The effects of cannabis vary from person to person, even if taking the same exact amount and type of cannabis. Several factors affect how a person reacts to cannabis. These factors include:

- Dosage (amount used)

- Environment or setting, including setting of cultivation, preparation, storage and use

- Strain of cannabis used and how it is consumed

- History and experience of cannabis use

- Mindset (mood) on consumption

- Biochemistry

- Nutrition or current diet

Hemp is the term used for the variety cultivated for fiber. This has smaller amounts of THC (psychoactive cannabinoid), typically not more than 1%, compared to other strains.

Chapter 9

How To Use Cannabis Root

The roots have high levels of CBD, which is a good characteristic. This compound has some therapeutic benefits without the psychoactive effects that the leaves and flowers provide. This is more appealing to a lot of people because the psychoactive effects can be unpredictable. At times, these psychoactive effects may hinder a person from functioning normally in their daily routine.

Cannabis roots may even be used to counter THC effects, like for someone who consumed excessive amounts of cannabis edibles with large amounts of THC.

CBD is least in the flowers (bud). The greater concentrations are found in the stems, leaves and roots. Of these, the roots have the highest CBD levels, acting as storage tanks of this therapeutic compound.

These roots can be used as the main therapeutic ingredient or to fortify extractions and infusions. It can be eaten raw or added to edibles such as smoothies and juices, even food like breads and stews. Drinking tea is one of most common ways to consume cannabis roots.

For smoothies, start with 2 teaspoons of root. Drink and wait for at least 1 hour for the CBD to kick in. observe how long it took for effects to start kicking in then monitor how long the effect lasted and what time the effects start to wane. Pain will disappear, leaving a relaxed feeling, without the typical heavy buzz associated with THC. The person will feel more energetic and pain-free for the rest of the day while still being able to perform daily activities.

There are many other ways to receive cannabis roots. These methods date back to thousands of years and remained pretty much the same. The root can be used raw, roasted, turned into ash, powdered, soaked, boiled or dried. In ancient times, ash of cannabis root mixed with honey is applied directly on the scalp for rejuvenating hair growth.

Boiling the roots or immersing in water in water makes tea. Boiling for extended periods creates a dark, thick extract that looks like heavy oil or pitch. Roasted or dried roots may be used as it is or ground into powder that can be mixed for poultices or salves. Soaking the roots in water and dipping a bandage in it creates a soothing compress that can help with irritated, burned or inflamed skin.

Chapter 10

Medicinal Cannabis Oil

Medicinal cannabis oil is prepared by using marijuana resin concentrate. This highly effective cannabis preparation can be used for treating all types of inflammation and pain. Cannabis oil contains large levels of CBD.

The CBD activates the CB2 receptors found in the body. These receptors play roles in controlling inflammatory process. They can effectively block the sensation of pain, too.

This oil is also rich in THC. In reduced doses, medicinal medical marijuana oil use also causes enhanced moods and feelings of well-being.

Strains to Use to Make Cannabis Oil

The best choice for making cannabis oil is the indica strain. Hybrids with indica dominance can also be used. These strains have high THC levels, as well as high CBD concentration. Examples include the Bubba Kush and the Critical Cheese seed strains. These can work for those who want the healing effects of cannabis on the physical level.

Sativa may also be used. Example strains are Strawberry Haze and Original Amnesia. These can work for those who want the cannabis oil to produce mood-lifting effects from the main alkaloid THC.

Types of Oil

There are many different types of oil extracted from the cannabis plant. Terms like hemp oil, cannabis oil, THC oil, CBD oil, and marijuana oil can be confusing. Are these the same and treat the same list of disorders or not?

These names typically refer to the same thing- oil extracted from the cannabis plant. The biggest difference is o the THC contents. CBD oil and hemp oil have almost negligible amounts of THC. Contents are almost non-existent. Other types of oil contain THC in varying measurable concentrations.

- Hemp oil

Hemp oil is also known as hemp seed oil. The seeds are a by-product of hemp fiber production.

Hemp oil is different from cannabis oil. Hemp oil is extracted from hemp, which are strains cultivated for use as fiber, not for medicinal purposes. This oil is typically low in THC but with higher CBD levels. Cannabis oil has a higher concentration of THC.

Cold-pressed hemp seed oil

Hemp seeds may be cold-pressed to extract the oils. The seeds may remain unpeeled or peeled prior to cold-press extraction. This oil has a delicious flavor. Its nutrient contents are great, with good amounts of unsaturated fats, including omega-3 and omega-6.

There are no CBD or THC present in these oils (both hemp oil and cold-pressed hemp seed oil). However, these can be added to other cannabis preparations to improve dosage. Hemp oil can also improve the effects of CBD oil when combined.

- CBD oil

CBD oil is extracted from fiber hemp. The difference with hemp oil is that CBD oil contains active cannabinoids. It at least has cannabidiol. Other bioactive compounds may also be present in minute amounts. There may be other cannabinoids such as CBC, CBDA, CBGA and CBCA. However, CBD oil does not have any THC.

CBD oil is often available diluted with hemp seed oil or olive oil. This kind of dilution helps improve the taste and the dosage of CBD oil.

CBD oil does not give the "high" that marijuana is known for. This is because the oil is obtained from hemp plant that naturally has low THC levels.

This oil is legally available in most places, especially in Europe. The absence of THC in this oil is one of the major reasons for its widespread use and availability. It is available in many different tastes and types, too.

- Marijuana oil

This type of oil is available in two forms- cannabis oil ad THC oil. These are basically derived from THC-rich cannabis (marijuana) plant strains. The most common being the Dutch marijuana. At times, marijuana oil, cannabis oil and THC oil are used interchangeably.

The primary purpose of taking these oils is for its psychoactive effects. In recent years, these oils are also increasingly being used for its medicinal effects.

The oil is typically created from the resin extracted from the female marijuana plant using alcohol as solvent. The resulting mixture is set aside to allow alcohol component to escape. The residue is a thick syrup with high THC concentrations, with significant CBD amounts as well. The syrup is diluted in pure hemp seed oil to make it easier for dosing and use.

The differences might be on the amount of THC present. All of these oils have high THC contents. THC oil has the highest concentration, as the name already suggests. Cannabis oil and marijuana oil have varying concentrations of THC.

These oils are not available to buy because of the THC content. THC is generally illegal although a few places have some form of legislation that regulates its production, purchasing, sale and use.

Advantages of Using Oils

Oils from the roots are better than smoking the flower for many reasons:

- Not breathing in carcinogens or other chemicals

- Allows for oral or topical use, and also in inhalation forms (i.e., vaporizers)

- Allows for more targeted treatment

- More potent than smoked flower

- Quicker relief

- Allows for more consistent dosing

- Available in more flavors

Uses of cannabis oil

The medicinal cannabis oil has pain relief, arterial tension relief and anti-inflammatory effects. These are mainly from the CBD effect. THC and the other cannabinoids also promote some health benefits. Therapeutic benefits may include:

- Mood improvement

- Skin cell regeneration

- Appetite stimulant

- Intraocular pressure reducer

- Decrease in frequency of occurrence of epileptic seizures

Chapter 11

Therapeutic benefits

The following therapeutic benefits are based in modern studies as well as anecdotal reports form users/

1. Reduce anxiety and stress

Cannabis oil can help in relaxing the mind and promote the release of the pleasure hormones. These effects help relieve high levels of stress and anxiety. A peaceful and calming feeling takes over after using the oils.

The cannabinoids activate the different specific receptors located at different areas in the body. This activation produces the pharmacologic effects on the immune system and central nervous system.

One study conducted in 2013 at Israel's University of Haifa demonstrated how cannabinoid treatment could help with trauma. People who experienced a traumatic event may be able to regulate their emotional responses to trauma. Stress-induced impairment typically associated with traumatic experiences is also reduced.

Cannabinoids were found to effectively minimize the stress receptors located in the basolateral amygdala. These are the nuclei receiving most of the sensory information. The stress receptors in the hippocampus are also reduced in cannabinoid treatment. The hippocampus is the brain area considered as the seat of emotions.

2. Insomnia

People suffering from insomnia may also benefit from cannabis oil. The calming effect helps promote better sleep quality.

One scientific review published in 2015, in the *American Journal of Health-System Pharmacy* presented that cannabis treatment can help those with PTSD. Veterans suffering from post-traumatic stress disorder found having less trouble falling and staying asleep. The research proposed that psychoactive components found in unrefined cannabis are able to regulate the release of neurotransmitters. This action results in a large variety of CNS effects. These include alteration of processes involved in memory and increase in pleasure. These help a person to deal with the negative impact of traumatic events.

Cross-sectional studies were also conducted. These studies found that there is a direct correlation between cannabis use and severe PTSD. Military veterans who underwent cannabis treatment reported reduced insomnia and anxiety, with improved coping abilities.

3. Altered appetite

People with poor appetite after injury recovery or illness may benefit from the appetite-stimulating effect of cannabis oil. It stimulates the digestive system and induce feelings of hunger. This is a result of hormonal stimulation caused by the presence of the cannabinoids.

One article in the *International Weekly Journal of Science*, states that cannabis can effectively stimulate the body to release certain hormones that promote hunger.

The nerves are also important in this process. There are neurons that promote hunger while there are those that suppress it. Hence, cannabis can both promote appetite and suppress it, depending on which neuron is activated.

These actions make cannabis a natural treatment for obesity and eating disorders. The cannabinoid system in the body (receptors that can interact with cannabinoids for therapeutic benefits) plays a central role in this event. More research on this interaction is ongoing to provide greater understanding and uncover more potential benefits.

4. Better eye health

A number of researches demonstrated that using cannabis oil could help in treating glaucoma and macular degeneration naturally. Glaucoma affects the optic nerve, resulting in the loss of vision that may lead to blindness. The damage is caused by increasing IOP (intraocular pressure) from fluid accumulation. Fluid builds up within the eyes and places undue pressure on the lens, retina and optic nerve.

If not treated immediately, this pressure can cause permanent damage to the affected eye structures.

The American Glaucoma Society conducted several studies. They found out that cannabis could help lower IOP. This is an indication that cannabis oil can be used in treating glaucoma naturally. However, the studies also found that the IOP-lowering effects are only short-lived. Cannabis oil would have to be used every 3 hours to sustain the effects.

Oil is not administered directly on the eyes. NEVER apply anything directly into the eyes unless it has been medically cleared to be an optic medication.

5. Pain relief

Cannabis is historically used for pain relief. Research found evidences indicating that cannabinoids plays a role in pain pathways. The cannabinoids inhibit the neuronal transmission of pain.

Cannabis oil is used for cancer patients who are undergoing chemotherapy. It helps alleviate inflammation and chronic pain. In the same manner, cannabis oil can be used as part of natural treatment for fibromyalgia.

6. Improve heart health

Cannabis oil has antioxidant properties that will benefit the heart and the rest of the cardiovascular system. These antioxidants help prevent the development of cardiovascular disease.

Animal studies found indications that the use of cannabis oil helps in preventing a wide range of conditions affecting the heart and blood vessels. These include coronary heart disease, heart attacks, stroke, hypertension, and atherosclerosis.

The University of Nottingham School of Medicine conducted a study in 2014 regarding cannabis effects on the blood vessels. This was the first human study to be conducted for cannabis. The result of the study suggested that cannabis could cause the relaxation of the blood vessels. This is an indication of a possibility of using cannabis as a natural treatment for lowering blood pressure. This effect could also help in improving circulation.

This is just the first study so far. More research is needed to confirm that cannabis can help improve cardiovascular health. More studies are also needed to prove that cannabis is a safe treatment for cardiovascular issues.

7. Skin protectant

Cannabis oil applied on the skin has a few benefits. It promotes faster skin cell turnover by speeding up shredding of dead skin cells. This helps in promoting the emergence of new, younger and healthier skin for a glowing, fresh and youthful looking skin.

The cannabinoids also promote lipid production within the skin. This action helps in regulating skin problems that involve over- or underproduction of oil, such as acne and dry skin.

Cannabis oil also helps with accelerated skin aging. Exposure to toxins, UV radiation and free radicals, cause cellular damage through the oxidation process. Oxidation speeds up the aging process and causes premature lines and wrinkles, as well as dry and dull skin. Cannabis oil has high antioxidant concentrations. This helps in combating and removing free radicals.

Consuming cannabis oil is also known to promote relaxation and reduce stress. Accelerated aging also results from chronic high levels of stress.

8. Cancer prevention

There is still a need for more conclusive evidence about the cancer-prevention effects of cannabis. So far, cannabis is still considered as part of natural cancer treatment and cancer prevention. The cannabinoids demonstrated ability to shrink tumors.

These compounds also help with the side effects of cancer treatment such as weakness, nausea, and lack of appetite.

The US FDA has not yet approved the use of cannabis for cancer treatment or for any other medical condition. However, research indicates the anti-cancer properties of cannabis.

In Canada, a case report was published in 2013. The benefits of cannabis oil on cancer were evaluated in a 14-year old female patient. The patient was diagnosed with ALL or acute lymphoblastic leukemia. The patient was severely underweight and extremely ill. All other treatment options were revoked, including aggressive chemotherapy, radiation therapy, and standard bone marrow transplant. Treatment was already considered failure for this patient.

There were no other conventional treatments available for this patient. The family turned to cannabis extracts. They administered extracts orally to the patient every day.

The cannabis administration started as a once daily dose, increasing gradually. By the 15th day, the patient was already receiving treatment three times a day. As the cannabis treatment progressed, the patient was slowly decreasing the use of morphine for pain. Alertness was increased. There were symptoms of euphoria and disoriented memory. All these are consistent with known effects of cannabis usage.

Treatment continued for 65 days. During the entire time, strains used were repeatedly changed. Some strains were effective in inducing better appetite and relieving pain.

The cannabis oil was diluted in hemp oil. Honey was mixed to improve the viscosity and bitter taste. Honey is a known natural digestive aid.

The patient experienced some marked improvements in terms of pain and appetite. This indicated that cannabis should be considered for cancer treatment. There is a need to further explore the effects of certain strains due to possibility of selective attack on cancer cells. Some strains may reduce the extensive cytotoxic effects of current conventional chemotherapeutic agents.

However, the patient eventually died due to bowel perforation and gastrointestinal bleeding.

This case study showed that blast counts were inadequately controlled by advanced chemotherapeutic agents. Blast counts are cells in the bone marrow and the blood. This failure resulted in devastating effects that resulted in the patient's death.

On the other and, the cannabis therapy did not result in any toxic side effects. It only had a few psychosomatic properties, some of which increased the patient's vitality.

These psychosomatic effects can be bypassed by using cannabis with non-psychoactive contents such as CBD. This still had significant anti-proliferative effects.

Cannabinoids inhibit tumor cell growth, as observed in cultures. Animal studies revealed that cannabinoids modulate the key cell signaling pathways of tumor proliferation. These are worth exploring, in a world where cancer is fast spreading and claiming more lives with each passing year.

Cannabis oil dose for cancer

The suggestion for taking cannabis oil for cancer is to take three doses every day. Doses are gradually increased over a few days until full therapeutic effect is obtained. Daily increase is suggested at 1 gram increment. Full treatment dose is considered to be at 90 days.

Cannabis Essential Oil

This is another form of cannabis oil that can be used for many therapeutic benefits. It is usually extracted from the leaves and buds via distillation method. However, there is also a good amount of essential oil that can be extracted from the roots. Extraction methods might require longer processing to remove the oils from the roots.

This is a green liquid, unlike the thick dark syrup base of cannabis oil. The essential oil is highly volatile compared to the thick, viscous resin base material of cannabis oil. However, the components of the essential oil are highly potent.

Contents of the essential oil include active organic compounds such as sesquiterpenes and monoterpenes. Aside from therapeutic uses, essential oil is also used in candles, perfumes, and soaps. This may also be used in some foods.

The main manufacturer and distributor of cannabis essential oil is from France and several other countries in Europe. Exportation outside Europe may pose a few problems from other countries. Cannabis in all or some forms may be prohibited in some countries.

Cannabis essential oil is highly concentrated. Tiny amounts are already enough to produce therapeutic effects.

Benefits of cannabis essential oil

The essential oil can also produce the same effects as cannabis oil such as:

- Relieve stress and anxiety
  Volatile compounds help ease the mind and reduce the impact of stress-inducing and anxiety-driving thoughts, emotions, moods, and feelings.
- Treat insomnia
  People tend to sleep better when their minds are at ease and their stress levels are low.
- Boost appetite
  Taking cannabis helps improve appetite in people who are recovering from a long bout with an illness. This help speed up recovery time and return to good health status.
- Relieve pain

The cannabis essential oil can be used in all types of pain, even in emergency pain situations. For example, it can be applied topically over a recently injured leg for immediate pain relief while waiting for medical attention.

- Prevent cancer
  This is yet to be concluded by more research results. On numerous occasions, cannabis essential oil exhibited anti-tumor properties such as inhibiting abnormal rapid growth that leads to tumor development.
- Improve heart health
  Volatile oils help improve the fats and lipids balance in the body. It can help reduce the negative impact of some of the fats. These volatile oils may also help in removing excess cholesterol from the systems. These oils can also help in stimulating the various antioxidant processes in the body to benefit the heart and the blood vessels.
- Protect the skin from psoriasis and eczema
  Topically or orally, cannabis essential oil can help protect the skin against accelerated aging. It promotes faster replacement of dead skin cells for younger, healthier skin structure.
- Treat glaucoma
  Older people are at an increased risk for glaucoma and macular degeneration. Cannabis use showed potential in reducing these risks.
- Relieve migraines and headaches
  Topical application of a few drops over the temples can help provide instant relief from migraines and headaches.

How to Use

Cannabis essential oil can be used in the same way as other herbal essential oils. It should be diluted in a carrier oil for easy dosing. The pure essential oil is highly concentrated and may cause some untoward side effects, like most other essential oils.

Carrier oils that can be used include hemp seed oil and olive oil. Cannabis essential oil can be applied topically or used orally.

Chapter 12

Cannabis Root Recipes

How to make cannabis root oil extract

1. Take a few pieces of cannabis roots. Clean thoroughly with large amounts of water. All dirt should be removed.

2. Let the roots dry naturally. Hang them to keep moisture from accumulating within the root system. Leave to dry for 1 week.

3. Take the dry roots and cut into smaller sections using a scissor. Or, grind up the dry roots in a food processor.

4. Mix oil and water in a small pan.

5. Add the ground or cut up roots.

6. Cook the mixture over slow fire for 14 hours.

7. Check regularly and add more water as needed. Never allow the mixture to dry out.

8. Strain the liquid after 14 hours.

9. Pour strained liquid in a new pan.

10. Squeeze the roots to get as much of the juice as possible.

11. Add the juice into the liquid in the new pan.

12. Let the liquid sit for a few minutes for the oil to separate from the water. After a few minutes, oil will start to form a layer on the surface.

13. Place the pan in the freezer. Leave it there for a few hours.

14. Check the mixture if the oil layer starts to solidify.

15. Take the pan out of the freezer.

16. Scrape out the hardened oil layer carefully so that no water will be removed along with the oil. This step will be easier if you wait for the water to turn to ice before removing the oil layer.

17. Place the oil layer in a glass bowl.

18. Leave at room temperature to turn into liquid state.

This is now ready for use in various preparations. This oil can be added to beeswax, coconut oil, olive oil, hemp seed oil, shea butter, other essential oils and other recipes to use in any way preferred.

To Make a Salve

1. Get a double boiler.

2. Place beeswax in the double boiler, about the size of a thumb.

3. Add the cannabis root oil.

4. Allow the beeswax to melt.

5. Stir the liquid together until well mixed.

6. Transfer the mixture in a new, clean glass container.

7. Allow to cool.

This salve is now ready for use. It can be used to soothe joint pains.

To increase the therapeutic effects (and aroma as well) of the salve, aromatic essential oil may be added. Examples are:

- Bergamot essential oil: for treatment of psoriasis and cold sores

- Neroli: to reduce and lighten stretch marks and scars

- Chamomile: for treatment of inflammation (skin, muscle, joint), dermatitis, and eczema

- Black pepper: for reducing symptoms of arthritis and relieving cramps and muscle aches

How to make infused oil

1. Get ground dried roots of cannabis and olive oil or coconut oil.

2. Place ground roots and oil in a crock pot. Pour enough oil to cover the ground root by 1-2 inches deep. How much dried root and oil depends on desired concentration of the infused oil. Adjust as desired.

3. Set the crock pot on very low heat.

4. Let the mixture gently heat up for 4 to 5 hours.

5. Turn off the heat.

6. Let the mixture cool down.

7. Once cool, strain the liquid and pour into sterilized dark-colored bottles.

To use infused oil:

The infused oil can be used in numerous ways. It can be added to food as flavor and for therapeutic benefits. It can be used topically. It can be added to soaps, lotions, creams or even shampoo.

It can be used to make a salve:

1. Mix 1 ounce beeswax and 8 ounces of infused oil in a double boiler.

2. Warm the mixture over low heat.

3. Heat until beeswax melts.

4. Remove from heat.

5. Add a few drops of essential oil such as peppermint, clove, cardamom, chamomile, bergamot, etc.

6. Add a small amount of vitamin E. This will serve as preservative to keep the oils from becoming rancid.

7. Gently stir to mix everything.

8. Pour the mixture into a glass jar.

9. Allow to cool at room temperature.

10. Check the consistency. Adjust the amount of beeswax according to preferred consistency of the salve. Add more beeswax for a thicker consistency. Reduce beeswax for a softer salve consistency.

11. To adjust, gently reheat the salve and add more beeswax (thicker) or more infused oil (softer consistency).

Here is another recipe for creating cannabis root salve:

1. Pour 2 cups of coconut oil in a pan. Heat gently until it melts. Set aside.

2. Measure 1 to 2 ounces of marijuana roots.

3. Cut up or roughly grind in a food processor.

4. Place in a baking dish and bake in a preheated 200F oven for 10 minutes. The roots should be crispy but not burnt.

5. Transfer the baked roots into the pan with the melted coconut oil.

6. Simmer the mixture over low heat for 1 to 2 hours. Longer simmering will produce a more concentrated liquid.

7. Stir the mixture as it simmers every 10 minutes or so.

8. Check that the mixture does not boil.

9. Turn off the heat.

10. Strain the mixture through paper coffee filter or cheesecloth. Strain again as necessary until the oil is free of any plant residue. Set aside in a clean glass container.

11. Melt 1 ounce of beeswax in a new saucepan set over low heat.

12. Add 5 ounces of the coconut oil-cannabis mixture.

13. Mix gently and allow to simmer until everything is mixed well.

14. Do not allow the mixture to boil.

15. Once mixed, remove from heat.

16. Quickly add 1 tablespoon Vitamin E oil and stir well.

17. If adding other essential oils, add together with the vitamin E oil.

18. Mix well.

19. Pour cannabis salve in storage containers.

20. Allow to cool at room temperature before covering.

21. Store in the refrigerator but do not freeze.

How to Make Cannabis Root Balm

This can also be used as topical treatment for aching muscles and joints.

1. Get 1 to 2 clean cannabis root balls. Chop into very fine pieces. It does not have to be powdered, though, just very small. Place in a pot.

2. Measure about 4 cups of coconut oil. Add to the pot.

3. Measure 1 to 2 cups of water. The amount of water should be half of the amount of oil to be used. Add into the pot with the roots and coconut oil.

4. Simmer covered over low heat for 12 to 14 hours.

5. Remove from heat and set aside for 6 to 10 hours.

6. Repeat simmering for the next 3 to 4 days. Simmer for 12-14 hours then rest for 6 to 10 hours.

7. Check the amount of water. Add more as necessary to keep the coconut oil from burning off.

8. Strain the mixture to remove the plant residue.

9. Pour into a glass container. Cool slightly before placing in the refrigerator for overnight.

10. Once the oil layer has hardened, poke a few holes and drain the water off.

11. Check the consistency by reheating everything until melted.

12. Strain again and refrigerate. Remove excess water.

13. Prepare a few ounces of beeswax, if desired. Adding beeswax will help keep the balm semi-solid and smoother to apply over the skin.

14. If adding beeswax, gently warm the oil mixture up in a double boiler. Add the beeswax. Add a few for a softer consistency and more if you want the balm to be a bit more solid. Heat only until the oils are mixed well.

15. Remove from heat.

16. Vitamin E oil and essential oils are added at this point.

17. Stir gently to mix well.

18. Pour into glass containers with tight lids.

19. Cool before storing in the refrigerator for longer shelf life.

Cannabis Root Balm with Herbs

Few strains of cannabis can be used to make salves or balms. Some strains work better when alone while some may be mixed with other strains. It takes a few trial and error episodes to see what works best.

Aside from different cannabis strains, other herbs may be mixed as well. Examples are cloves, cinnamon, and anise. These can be added to increase the usefulness of the balm and to be able to treat a wider range of ailments. These added herbs may also help in improving the scent of the balm.

Before the root is made into balm, it is typically dried first. This helps increase the storage life. The moisture from the roots may become breeding ground for bacteria and fungi. This may also cause the balm to go rancid faster.

1. Dry the roots well under the sun for a few days. Some place the roots in a mesh bag and hang it to air dry.

2. After the roots are dried, it is cut up into smaller pieces. Place in a food processor or blender and pulse until the dried roots turn into rough powder. The roots may also be ground using a mortar and pestle.

3. Place the rough root powder in a slow cooker. Add some oil and water. Adding water keeps the mixture from drying out. Without water, the oil will fry the root powder. Check that the mixture contains enough water. Add more water as necessary to keep the mixture from drying out.

4. Gently heat up the mixture for up to 12 hours. Slow heating will release volatile compounds from within the root and mix with the oil. These volatile compounds include terpenoids and some cannabinoids.

5. After heating for about 12 hours, strain the liquid off. The root pulp is strained out. This may be discarded. The root pulp may also be frozen for another processing, but up to two times of use. Otherwise, the balm will lose a significant amount of active healing compounds.

6. Place the liquid in the freezer. The water freezes while volatile oils float to the surface. This makes it easier to separate the oil. At this point, the oil will be semi-solid with a waxy consistency. Once it is placed at room temperature, the oil will turn liquid with a translucent, smooth appearance.

7. Place the separated oil in a small saucepan.

8. Reheat gently over very low fire.

9. Add beeswax, enough so that the oil is less runny.

10. The product should have a more spreadable consistency even at room temperature.

How to Make Cannabutter (Cannabis Butter)

This can be used for cooking or flavoring foods while enjoying the therapeutic benefits.

1. Prepare ¼ ounce of finely ground cannabis root.

2. Get one stick or ½ cup of unsalted butter.

3. Melt the butter in a saucepan set over low heat.

4. Add ground cannabis root, small amounts at a time.

5. Stir to mix well.

6. Simmer the mixture for 45 minutes, frequently stirring to keep the bottom from burning. Small bubbles should appear on the surface as the mixture simmers and not large ones. Do not allow the mixture to boil. The butter might get burned.

7. Strain the butter to remove the ground roots.

8. Press a spoon over the ground roots in the strainer to squeeze out any remaining cannabis extract and butter.

Root Tea

This is one of the easiest to prepare. This has been well documented in the ancient Chinese text by Emperor Shen Nung.

Therapeutic effects of cannabis root tea include:

- Respiratory obstructions

- Menstrual pain

- Pain from surgery involving the internal organs

- Asthma

- Internal hemorrhage

To make root tea:

1. Clean the roots very well. Remove all dirt.

2. Cut the roots into smaller chunks.

3. Grinding the roots into powder.

4. Leave on a shallow container to dry out completely.

5. Take a small amount of root powder.

6. Add to a pot with a liter of water.

7. Boil over medium high heat.

8. Strain and pour into a cup.

9. It's ready to drink.

Never use roots that have been treated or exposed to chemicals. These contain harmful toxins that produce more negative effects.

The tea is potent and can help treat certain ailments. However, it is not recommended to be taken on daily. Excessive and long term intake may cause some problems, such as some damage to the blood.

Chapter 13

Potential Risks

Cannabis roots have a huge potential as a treatment option for numerous diseases. One important thing to remember in the use of cannabis root is hepatotoxicity. The active compounds may damage the liver if taking high doses of cannabis roots.

The most likely to cause damage to the liver are the compounds piperidine and pyrrolidine. These alkaloids may also irritate the lining of the stomach. This is why drinking cannabis root tea has a higher risk for side effects and discomforts than when using topically.

However, these same alkaloids are also known to irritate the lungs, mucus membranes and skin. Care and constant monitoring for responses are important in order to make the necessary adjustment in dose.

Studies show that these alkaloids are not found in amounts large enough to pose a serious risk. However, prolonged, and excessive use should be avoided.

Cannabis root extract must not be taken in pure, undiluted form.

Long-term consumption of tea may not have any serious risk. Regular consumption should be only light to moderate.

For topical use, monitor responses while in use. If any reaction appears at any point of topical treatment, discontinue use. Untoward reactions from topical use typically stop when the use of topical cannabis root is discontinued. There are no known long-term ill effects from topical use.

Definitive toxicity levels or potential risks are yet to be established through more research. The use of cannabis for medical treatment is still in its infancy stage.

Safety with use is of primary importance. So far, it is highly recommend to take small doses and for short-term treatment. At any time that any untoward reactions appear, discontinue use immediately and seek medical help.

Chapter 14

Safe Consumption Guidelines

Safety with use is a priority with all forms of cannabis for all purposes. It is important to know and understand the different methods of taking cannabis for medical purposes.

- Ingestion through eating

Eating cannabis is one of the safest methods to take it for medical purposes. The effects can be experienced to a greater degree than when taking it in inhalation form. The onset of the effects is delayed but lasts longer. Delay of onset is typically about an hour or so compared to the onset when taking via inhalation.

It takes a few experimentations with edible cannabis before the right dose and type is determined for a particular health concern.

Digestion of cannabinoids also changes the way these compounds are metabolized. Effects would be differently subjective, based on individual digestive and metabolic processes.

Use only small amounts of edibles initially. Wait for 2 hours and evaluate responses. If response is good and no negative side effects are felt, increase doses if necessary. Increase should be gradual and continuous monitoring of responses should be done when finding the right dose. Excessive doses easily occur with edibles. This can make the experience very uncomfortable.

Ways to eat cannabis includes using cannabis oil or hash. Some also use sprays or tinctures.

For tinctures and sprays, do not exceed two drops on initial use. Wait for an hour and check for response. If no untoward side effects are experienced, dose may be increased gradually, as needed.

- Application via topicals

This is one of the safest ways to take cannabis. This also has the least risk for serious side effects. Psychoactive effects are also at the least, because absorption and effect tends to be localized only to the treated area. Topicals are the best options for direct relief for several ailments or pains.

- Inhalation via smoking

This method produces quick results. Inhalation through smoking cannabis is the quickest way to provide relief. Finding the best individual dose is still based on a trial and error process.

According to research, smoking cannabis does not pose an increased risk for lung cancer or other types of cancer. However, this method still poses risks for bronchial issues like harsh cough. This is from inhaling potential irritants such as tar.

To reduce these risks, smoke minimally. Start with 1-3 inhalations. Wait for about 10 to 15 minutes and evaluate response. Gradually increase to get the relief needed. Note the dosage and form used as reference for future dosing.

When smoking cannabis, take shallow, small inhales instead of deep ones. Studies show that holding the smoke within the lungs will not produce a significantly greater effect. Hence, shallow inhales are enough. In fact, a majority of active THC, around 95%, are already absorbed within the first few seconds of inhalation.

It is highly advisable to avoid using lighters and matches to light up the cannabis. This is to avoid contaminating cannabis with chemicals from these lighting materials. A better alternative is to use hemp paper coated with beeswax.

- Inhalation via vaporizer

This is widely considered as the safest method in inhaling cannabis medication. The cannabis-containing oil is heated until it becomes vapors. The vapors carry the active cannabinoids and leave behind other plant material that may cause side effects. This form also reduces the amount of chemical irritants like tar that may be inhaled. Odor is also much less from vaporizers compared to other types of smoking.

- Inhalation via steam roller/one-hitter/pipe

Choose brass, stainless steel or glass pipes. Using plastic or wooden pipes will affect the flavor, quality and dose received from inhaling cannabis. The heat may also cause wood or plastic material to burn or heat up and release some contaminants.

There are available glass one-hitters. These are tubular pipes that carry single doses. These are the most methods available for inhaling cannabis.

- Inhalation via water pipe/bong

This is another method of consuming cannabis but is not recommended for regular use. There is a tendency that water drops or water vapors will be inhaled into the lungs.

Do not use bongs made from aluminum, rubber, or plastic. These materials may melt or may produce harmful fumes.

Change the water frequently. Fungi, molds, viruses, and bacteria may grow on water left in the bong or water pipe for a long time.

Tips to Determining the Right Strain and Dose

People react to the different varieties of cannabis differently. The therapeutic dose will differ from person to person because of the individual factors such as metabolic rate, health and so on. Hence, getting the right dose and the appropriate strain or hybrid for specific medical purposes would require a few experimentations.

Here are a few tips on how to find the right strain and dose:

1. Record reactions to every variety tried. This includes variety (if hybrid, note dominant strain), form (e.g., hashish, oil, edible, etc.), dose, mode of consumption (e.g. eating, inhaling, etc.), therapeutic effects (e.g., relieved muscle spasms, reduced nausea, etc.), and side effects, if any.

2. Try starting with more concentrated forms. This will help in controlling doses better, allowing for use of much smaller amounts and easy dose tracking. Working with cannabis concentrate is easier when higher doses are needed. For example, it is easier to monitor taking a few concentrated drops of cannabis oil than eating a dozen of cannabis edibles.

3. A glass pipe should be used solely for cannabis concentrates. This makes it easier to control the doses.

4. Try various cannabis strains. Do not be afraid to work with high CBD contents. These are typically effective for pain, nausea and appetite.

5. Schedule medicine vacation. Long term, continued use is not recommended. Cannabis does not promote tolerance like opiates. Effects tend to be enhanced when cannabis use is restarted. Stop use or reduce intake for as long as desired.

6. Even after finding the right variety and dose, monitor response. If the current variety seems to be losing its effectiveness, try another strain or another form.

7. Organic cannabis products should be used as much as possible. This reduces nasty side effects from contaminants like pesticides and artificial fertilizers. Never take cannabis treated or exposed to pesticides. It's toxic.

Drug Interactions

At this time, there are no negative interactions reported between cannabis and other drugs. Some studies did find that cannabis enhances the action of opiate painkillers. There is little information on the interaction between cannabis and other pharmaceutical drugs. Despite that, it is still imperative to monitor for any complimentary effects.

Before taking cannabis to treat any health issue, it is best to consult with a doctor. People taking medication therapies should work with their doctor for safety of use.

There are some studies that showed cannabis may interact with fluoxetine, antihistamines, disulfiram, theophylline, sedatives, and barbiturates.

Mixing alcohol and cannabis can create a synergistic effect. This means that each enhances the effect of the other. Limit the use of these together or within a few hours of taking of one or the other.

Safety Precautions

Safety of use extends not only in proper dosing. It extends on precautions to take before, while and after use.

- Avoid operating heavy machineries, driving or doing anything that requires alertness when taking *C. indica* strain and indica-dominant hybrids. This strain can cause a person to become drowsy.
- Driving is highly discouraged when taking cannabis, in any form, with any strain or hybrid. Cannabis can impair a person's motor skills a few hours after consumption. Before driving, wait for about 1 to 2 hours after medicating to reduce risks for accidents.

Keeping Track of Cannabis Use

Optimal treatment results from balancing doses, mode of intake and type of strain used. Record the entire treatment period to keep track of what is effective and what produces the greatest therapeutic effect. This will be an important evaluation tool to determine if cannabis use is effective or if adjustments need to be made. This is especially so when cannabis is used in conjunction with other therapies, such as chemotherapy.

A detailed log for at least 1 week is already very helpful. Here are the things that the log should at least contain:

- Date/Time: Always note down date and time of cannabis consumption.

- Amount: Write down how much cannabis used every time. Either place the gram estimate or other forms of consistent measure such as teaspoon.

- Strain: Note the name, variety or strain of the cannabis used as medicine. If the name is not available, provide a detailed description of the cannabis medicine.

- Code: The strains may be described in codes. For example, S=Sativa, I=Indica, I/S= Indica-dominant Sativa Cross and S/I=Sativa-dominant Indica Cross.

- Type: This refers to the consumed form of cannabis. This includes dried bud flower (most common), tincture/sprays, concentrates, topical or edibles/drinks. Codes may also be used for this to make it easier to note down and remember: F=flower, T=tincture/spray, C=concentrate, TO=topical, E=edible

- Cannabinoid Content: This refers to the concentration of cannabinoids such as CBD, THC and/or CBN. Write the percentages of each if information is available. If not, at least note down the preparation and potency.

- Mode: Note how the medication was used. Codes for the type of se may be used: TO=topical, V=vaporize or S=smoke, T=tincture or spray, E=eat/digest

- Therapeutic Effects: Write any positive effects experienced after taking cannabis. Include all therapeutic effects such as physical, social, mental, behavioral, etc.

- Negative Side Effects: List any negative effects, such as if there was burning or irritation when using topicals for eczema, harsh cough after 2 inhalation, etc.

- Timing: Monitor the time from the moment the cannabis is taken up to the moment the therapeutic benefits started to be felt. For example, note down the time when the cannabis cream was applied on the psoriatic skin area and note how long it took before the itching and inflammation started to lessen.

Monitoring does not stop there.

Continue observing when the peak effects were felt. In the same example, note down when the pain relief started to be felt then continue monitoring when pain was no longer there.

Continue monitoring.

Note the time when the therapeutic effects started to wane.

Lastly, note the time when all the effects are no longer evident.

Other things that can be noted down include:

- Reason for cannabis use

Write the specific factors that prompted use. For example, there is itchiness, inflammation, and pain over eczematous skin area or overwhelming nausea, anxiety, and so on.

- Mindset

Write the feelings and mood before and after cannabis use.

- Setting

Document the conditions surrounding the time of using cannabis. Take note of the place, possibly the temperature (hot, cold, humid, windy, etc.), and position (standing, lying down, sitting, reclining, etc.)

- Companions

It is also important to note if with other people at the time when the cannabis as consumed.

- Activities

Observe and note down the activities before using cannabis. If possible, write the events that led to the use. For example, walking outside and smelled grilled pork when nausea was experienced.

Chapter 15

Marijuana Laws in the United States

The first state-level legislation passed in the United States that legalized medical use of marijuana was in 1996, in the state of California. In the following years, 22 states with Guam and the District of Columbia legislated some form of laws allowing for medical use of marijuana. More states are also on the road to creating their own laws regarding medical marijuana.

Details of these laws vary among the states. The general conditions are that these laws allow people to procure marijuana for their symptoms provided they have a physician's order for the use of marijuana. Conditions that may use marijuana for symptom alleviation range from social anxiety to glaucoma.

The legalization for medical use of cannabis or marijuana divided the society. Some are fervently against it while some are thankful for the laws. Despite the divide, the path towards cannabis legalization is unique in the history of America on medical and drug policies.

Despite the state laws, cannabis in all its forms (both recreational and medical) remains treated as illegal under the federal law.

Marijuana Under Federal Laws

Marijuana was first regulated by the federal government in 1937. Congress at that time passed the Marijuana Tax Act. This was patterned after the earlier Congress bill in 1914 called the Harrison Narcotic Act. This particular act by the Congress regulated and taxed drugs instead of outright prohibition. This made it less at risk for any legal challenges in the future. The Harrison Narcotic Act regulated and taxed heroin, morphine and similar drugs. In this form, these drugs were essentially prohibited in effect.

Marijuana Tax Act operated in the same way. It was supposedly a revenue measure but the effect was the prohibition of sale or possession of marijuana.

After the 1937 Act, tougher measures were created. One example was the 1952 Boggs Act. This provided strict mandatory sentences for any offense that involved marijuana and other similar kinds of drugs.

The Controlled Substances Act in 1970 was passed by Congress. This established the schedules or categories of individual drugs based on potential for abuse and supposed medical usefulness.

Substances under Schedule 1 were the most restricted ones. According to the federal government, these medications are considered to have no medical use. These also have the highest potential for abuse.

Under the Controlled Substances Act, as part of the war on drugs by President Nixon's, marijuana was classified under Schedule 1. Other substances classified in this category were LSD and heroin. This classification was believed to be more due to the animosity of Nixon on the counterculture associated with marijuana use. It was not mainly based on legal, medical or scientific opinion.

In 1972, Nixon appointed an investigative body called the Shafer Commission. The commission report suggested that marijuana should be decriminalized. The recommendation also included that marijuana should be removed from the Schedule 1 category.

Nixon passionately rejected the Commission's recommendations. Marijuana remained in this category.

Under the Schedule 1 category, it was difficult to have access to marijuana, even by scientists for research purposes. Hence, the potential for developing cannabis for medical use was seriously hampered. Standard protocols for scientific, medical and pharmaceutical studies were not applied to determine if there is or there isn't any medical use.

Despite the restrictions, marijuana is still available in a few select dispensaries. However, because of the restrictions and very few research and standards, marijuana from dispensaries was not consistent in dose, quality or strength. These were not manufactured with scientific standards. The strengths were not a result of scientific, rigorous, peer-reviewed controlled studies. Hence, there were inconsistent effects and reactions.

The Movement for Legalization

The drive towards legalization for marijuana originated from citizen support, not from the medical or pharmaceutical community. The citizen support came from state level, expressed through activism, ballot initiatives and lobbying.

The state interest on marijuana decriminalization and medical access started in the 1970s. During this decade, Maine, Alaska and Oregon decriminalized marijuana. In 1978, New Mexico passed legislation that allowed for a short-lived research program for medical marijuana.

States Currently Allowing Marijuana for Medical Use

Recent movements and growing evidences on potential medical use led to a few states allowing access to cannabis or marijuana. These states are:

- Arizona

- Alaska

- California

- Connecticut

- Colorado

- District of Columbia

- Delaware

- Hawaii

- Georgia

- Illinois

- Montana

- Maryland

- Maine

- Massachusetts

- Minnesota

- Michigan

- Nevada

- New York

- New Jersey

- New Hampshire

- New Mexico

- Oregon

- Texas

- Rhode Island

- Washington

- Vermont

Most of these states do not allow local stores to sell cannabis like selling cold medicines. Most of the legislations allow for use of cannabis with a doctor's prescription. Access is limited. There should be proof of illness or injury and a doctor's note or prescription before cannabis can be purchased.

State Laws

California was the first state to legalize the medical marijuana use in 1996.

To date, there are 44 states that allow cannabis use in some form. These state laws differ from each other. Some states allow for growing one's own marijuana for one's own use. Some states have laws that allow for sale of marijuana only if there is a medical proof and a doctor's prescription.

Some states, particularly Colorado, allow the use of marijuana for recreational purposes. In this state, anyone over 21 years old can simply walk into a store and purchase marijuana. Available forms range from seedlings to joints, to oils, and hashish. Some local shops even offer a huge selection of cannabis edible from classic pot brownies to gummy bears and even some creative ones like popsicles, beverages, candies and chocolate bars. There are also a huge selection of handcrafted cannabis-infused products such as soaps and numerous topicals. Even non-residents and tourists can have access and use of cannabis within Colorado State boundaries.

Alaska also has similar laws that allow for recreational use of marijuana. The state passed this legislation in 2014 via a ballot initiative.

Some states retain some restrictions.

Here is a summary of the different states and their general state view on marijuana use:

- Recreational use of marijuana allowed in

    o Alaska

    o Colorado

    o California

    o District of Columbia

    o Massachusetts

    o Maine

    o Oregon

    o Nevada

    o Washington

- Medical

- Arkansas
- Arizona
- Connecticut
- Florida
- Delaware
- Hawaii
- Louisiana
- Illinois
- Maryland
- Minnesota
- Michigan
- Montana
- New Jersey
- New Hampshire
- New Mexico
- North Dakota
- New York
- Ohio
- Rhode Island
- Pennsylvania
- West Virginia
- Vermont

- Limited Medical
  - Alabama
  - Iowa

- Indiana

- Missouri

- Georgia

- Kentucky

- Mississippi

- North Carolina

- South Carolina

- Oklahoma

- Tennessee

- Utah

- Texas

- Virginia

- Wyoming

- Wisconsin

- Prohibition

  - Kansas

  - Idaho

  - South Dakota

  - Nebraska (decriminalized)

Federal Laws

The federal government considers marijuana or cannabis as an illegal substance. There were a number of instances when federal laws on marijuana came in conflict with state laws.

In 2016, guidelines and policy memorandums were released by several federal agencies. These were attempts to manage the conflicts regarding medical marijuana.

The Department of Justice released a guidance memo about the enforcement of marijuana laws under the CSA or Controlled Substances Act. This memo was issued to prosecutors in August 2013. States should follow these guidelines when drafting, passing and enforcing their own marijuana laws

In this guidance memo, regulations for medical cannabis programs should follow these directives:

- No marijuana distribution to minors

- Revenue from marijuana sale must not benefit criminal gangs, cartels or enterprises

- No diversion of marijuana from states where it is legal to other states. For instance, marijuana is legal in Colorado but only within state borders. The marijuana from Colorado should not be delivered to other states or taken out of the state of Colorado.

- The state must ensure that state-authorized marijuana activities will not be used as pretext or cover for illegal activities such as trafficking other illegal drugs.

- The state must ensure that use of firearms or violence will not be involved in the cultivation and distribution of cannabis.

- Adverse consequences on public health resulting from marijuana use should be prevented, such as instituting measured against drugged driving

- Public lands must not be used for cultivating marijuana. Measures must be enforced to ensure the attendant dangers to the environment and public safety presented by marijuana cultivation.

- Possession and use of marijuana in federal properties must be prevented.

Conclusion

Again, thank you for downloading this book.

Cannabis has a long history of use. today, even after decades of debates ad numerous studies, cannabis remains to be a controversial herb.

The growing number of research and the increased awareness of the benefits may soon change the way society view cannabis.

I hope this book helped you gain a better understanding of cannabis.

If you decide to use cannabis for medicinal purposes, the information from this book will be your guide to becoming a responsible and accountable user.

Thank you.

Good luck!

www.ingramcontent.com/pod-product-compliance
Lightning Source LLC
Chambersburg PA
CBHW071121280526
45787CB00003B/1126